Dedication

To my beautiful wife

Table Of Contents

Introduction

Sugar comes in all forms, sizes, shapes and even hides itself in pastas, syrups, white rice, sodas and even bread. It impacts your body in negative way. Did you know that sugar is not a food group? Here's a few facts about sugar:

• Sugar contains no protein, healthy fats

• Sugar has no nutrients and vitamins

• Sugar contains no enzymes

Sugar is just an empty calories that can be very quickly digested and are responsible for pulling out vitamins from your body during digestion process. It does more harm than good. It's proven that your body - your temple has no physiological need for sugar, is it really worth it to get instant gratification?

Sugar in its most natural form is not harmful to the body, it's found naturally in fruits and vegetables. There are many forms of sugar such as *sucrose, dextrose* and *fructose.*

Chapter 1

Identifying Factors and Triggers

"There are two types of pain you will go through in life, the pain of discipline and the pain of regret. Discipline weighs ounces while regret weighs tons. "

- Jim Rohn

For you to be able to quit an addiction you have to identify the cause that drives you to engage in it, lucky for you, I have done numerous researches in that area!

We humans are driven by **2 basic mechanisms** that are rooted deeply in our brains:

- The desire to gain pleasure.
- The desire to avoid pain.

Okay, if it's so basic and simple, how come so many people are unable to stop themselves from consuming large quantities of sweets? Unfortunately, it's not that simple, for you to overcome this you'll have to reprogram your brain to dealing with pain and pleasure in a method that will benefit you in the long run instead of it amplifying the pain.

Programming the mind requires some time and actual application of the following steps, any failure upon your part in applying those steps will have its consequences as you'll see in the following chapter.

This chapter's main purpose is to identify and minimize the triggers and eliminate the environment that drives you to sabotage your progress or even get started!

Pick a pen and a sheet of paper and answer the following:

1. Under which circumstances do you tend to eat unhealthy sweets?
2. How do you rationalize the action?
3. You actually have inner conversations thorough the day without even noticing it!

What are the things you tell yourself right before eating junk sweets that minimize the pain of eating them and maximize the pleasure?

4. Under which emotional state do you consume these sweets?

5. What can you do right now to avoid getting into such lousy states?
6. What are the possible excuses you might come up with in the future to rationalize eating sweets?

What would you tell yourself when a friend tells you to take it easy and have a bite or two? When you're starving and you have a chocolate bar laying there?

Following though and writing down all the possible answers to these questions guarantees you'll start experiencing some cognitive dissonance while craving for unhealthy sweets!

These questions mark the answers to the core of your current addiction and by taking those questions on you're one step closer to making things happen!

Read the following tips ONLY after you complete the given tasks.

Tips and possible answers to these questions based on my experience:

- **Possible answers to question # 1:**

Family meetings, holidays and hangouts with your friends your time alone, having to do a task you don't consider fun.

- **Possible answers to question # 2:**

"I'm not losing weight anyways" ,"I tried this before and failed", "Christmas is right around the corner, I'll just enjoy it this one-time thing", "I can't let my family and friends down with a onetime request", "I only live once ,I should just enjoy it"

- **Possible answers to question #3:**

The main emotions you experience mostly before consuming sweets are painful emotions such as: anger, frustration, depression, regret, inadequacy. Sugar serves as a temporary anesthetic to the pain and the reason I said temporary is because they inflict you with heavy strokes of remorse afterwards.

- **Possible answers to question #4:**

This is a pretty good question that has many aspects to be addressed, this goes beyond mere addiction to junky sweets. It could possibly mean you having to stop hanging around certain people who are comfortable with an unhealthy lifestyle, change many of your current habits that lead you to that state! And maybe, just maybe, take your commitment to the next level by going for a daily walk.

- **Possible answers to question #5:**

"It gives me energy, why not?", "it can help me bulk and add muscle mass, sweets are high in calories in general", "It helps me to perform better", "It tastes better than any other healthy choice out there".

"We are what we repeatedly do, excellence, therefore is not an act, but a habit"

\- Aristotle

Summary of Chapter 1

Humans are driven by **2 basic mechanisms**:

- The desire to gain pleasure.
- The desire to avoid pain.

Pick a pen and a sheet of paper and answer these questions:

- Under which circumstances do you tend to eat unhealthy sweets?
- How do you rationalize the action?
- You actually have inner conversations thorough the day without even noticing it!
- Under which emotional state do you consume these sweets?
- What can you do right now to avoid getting into such lousy states?
- What are the possible excuses you might come up with in the future to rationalize eating sweets?

Chapter 2

Know Your Outcome!

"In order to succeed, your desire for success should be greater than your fear of failure."

- Bill Cosby

In this chapter you'll get to know why you have to take control of this kind of addiction and tame your desire:

    • Lots of sugar causes excessive amounts of insulin to be dumped in your blood.

Insulin is a storage hormone it boosts both muscular and fat synthesis.

There are 2 main types of carbs we'll be focusing on: *slow releasing and fast releasing.*

    Fast releasing carbs are mainly from junkie sweets and white carbohydrates, which are rapidly absorbed by the body and are easily stored as fats. Slow releasing are mainly -most vegetables, fruits such as yams, sweet potatoes, brown rice, are slowly digested and absorbed into your bloodstream, they do not cause your insulin to spike and therefore they feed your body for a longer period of time, keeping you full with minimal tendency to store fats.

Basically, eating lots of sweets and fast digesting carbs (fast releasing) can cause major fat storage that will result in extreme obesity.

There is plenty of research linking acidic blood pH and cancer (PH is a measurement of Acidity-Alkalinity in your blood, I encourage your to check Wikipedia if you want to know more detailed info about it). Cancer cells grow and thrive in an acidic environment and cannot survive in an alkaline environment.

Cancer cells produce lactic acid making your body even more therefore if you have cancer, your pH levels are lower than 7. 35 - ideal ph. level, and your body is too acidic.

Taking action to make your body more alkaline is vital in the battle against cancer.

So unless you have been eating a very healthy diet, full of fresh fruit and vegetables chances are good your body is too acidic, providing the perfect environment for cancer to grow. As your blood starts becoming acidic, your body deposits toxic acidic substances into cells to allow the blood to remain slightly alkaline which causes your cells to become more acidic and toxic, which results in a decrease of their oxygen levels, and harms their DNA and respiratory enzymes.

These dead cells themselves turn into acids. However, some of these acidified cells may adept in that environment. In other words, instead of dying as normal cells do in an acidic environment some cells survive by becoming abnormal cells.

These abnormal cells are called malignant cells and those cells do not correspond with brain function nor with our own DNA memory code.

Therefore, malignant cells grow indefinitely and without order thereby becoming what is known as cancer.

• From a different point of view, the link between PH levels and cancer is determined by the oxygenation of your cells.

• Alkaline water, including the water in cells, contains a lot of oxygen.

• Acidic water holds little to no oxygen.

• The more acidic your cells are, the less oxygenated they will be.

To make matters worse, the fermentation process cancer cells use to produce energy creates lactic acid, further increasing acidity and reducing oxygen levels.

Basically, when you over-eat sugary foods, you'll have to compensate for that by moving, breathing deeper and possibly go for a walk. Even that is not enough to reduce the sugar overload if you happen to consume large amounts of glucose.

If you're feeling intimidated after reading this, that's totally normal, I gradually discovered the truth, frankly, I only found out about the acidic- alkalinity/ PH and cancer relation this year and this info I have shared above helped me overcome my chocolate addiction and quitting many sugary candies and ice-creams.

The truth will set us free from the shackles we impose upon our minds, bodies and spirits. This is what happens when you keep eating sugary foods, you may research it yourself and read as many articles and books as you wish so that you'd be a 100% certain, I am not exaggerating.

Cause many people will tell you: "you are exaggerating" when you present them with the truth, you're not exaggerating, you happen to have a long term-long run sight which you live by and I salute you that!

Insulin is a storage hormone it boosts both muscular and fat synthesis.

There are 2 main types of carbs:
- *slow releasing*
- *fast releasing.*

Taking action to make your body more alkaline is vital in the battle against cancer.

When you over-eat sugary foods, you'll have to compensate for that by moving, breathing deeper and possibly go for a walk. Even that is not enough to reduce the sugar overload if you happen to consume large amounts of glucose.

Chapter 3

Getting Your Attitude Right

"The difference between a successful person and others is not a lack of strength, not a lack of knowledge, but rather a lack of will."

- Vince Lombardi

Have you tried committing to something before?
Quitting something for once and for all?

Have you managed to quit? Or have you had relapses and actually quit on quitting what's no longer serving you?
Life responds to deserve and not need, guess what? So do you.

You're never going to have what you truly want unless you truly know within your mind that you absolutely deserve it, the most important and the deceptive part knowing WHY you deserve it.

Before we move on I'd like you to answer those questions sincerely and honestly.
I want you to grab a pen and a paper and answer the following:

- Why do you want to quit eating junk sugary food?
- Why is it an absolute necessity and a must for you to undergo this process and conquer it?
- Why have you failed at quitting bad habits before?
- What would happen if you won't commit fully to this process? Which certain event triggered you to want to break this habit?

Possible answers and tips:

- After what you've read on chapter 2, you certainly want to live longer and enjoy the benefits of a better health, it's a noble purpose to want to live longer, serve this world and be around for those who you care for.

Maybe you want to shed some fat off? Look better & have more energy and vitality?

- It's an absolute must for you to go through this process because it will grow and develop your character to be the version you have to be in order to attain all that you wish for. It could be one of your core values to be in total control of your life and I truly understand that, wanting to make the best out of life while expanding and constantly improving your mindset and way of life.

- Possibly and most likely, never truly making up your mind while rationalizing doing the habit you're trying to break over and over again.

What's going on is that momentarily before engaging into sabotaging habits you tend to rationalize the pleasure they guarantee and minimize the pain they give to a point you're almost certain that it's a 100% pleasurable then the guilt kicks in before you start doing it but your mind goes like "Oh, what the hell, we're already at it" and guess what happens. **We fall back.**

- If you don't follow through and make sure you have your addictions in control they'll control you, you'll be their slave, mentally, emotionally and physically.
  You'll end up fat, with no energy or vitality; this could rob you and your family the joy of a lifetime and prevent you from experiencing life to its fullest. You'd be too lazy to do any form of physical activity, your low energy will prevent you from focusing in any type of activity, your work could deteriorate and your career could be on stake and if you're a family man or woman, we both know what follows next.

- Somebody telling you you're overweight? You found out today' 3 morning your pants were too tight for you even though you recently purchased them?

You found out you had diabetes? Somebody you know has cancer or had died from cancer?

Summary of Chapter 3

Please answer the following questions:

- Why do you want to quit eating junk sugary food?
- Why is it an absolute necessity and a must for you to undergo this process and conquer it?
- Why have you failed at quitting bad habits before?
- What would happen if you won't commit fully to this process?
- Which certain event triggered you to want to break this habit?

You're never going to have what you truly want unless you truly know within your mind that you absolutely deserve it, the most important and the deceptive part knowing WHY you deserve it.

Chapter 4

Forming a New Habits

A journey of a thousand miles begins with a single step
- Lao Tzu

Building the new is the most important part of the journey, getting into what's going to serve you long term is the name of the game.

Let's start our journey!

- Make sure there is the least possible amount of unhealthy junk sugary foods in your house.

- That includes your fridge and all of the closets.

- No soft drinks, no frozen pizzas, no chocolate, etc.

Get the better healthier alternative, experiment with what you like best.
The healthier alternative would be fruits and vegetables, fresh ones, no dried sugary fruit.

You need to eat fresh fruit and vegetables simply because they not only contain the highest quality of sugars (mainly fructose + bit of glucose) but they are also high in fiber which enhances your digestion and they simply energize you much more than any sugary snack or even coffee!

Eat lots of green vegetables, they are full of alkalinity which your body needs to balance your blood's PH and maintain perfect acidity levels.
I recommend getting a shaker/ juicer and making some vegetable green juice!
Recommended ingredients: cucumbers, lettuce, broccoli, celery and more veggies of your own personal preference.

Get in the gym and **commit to more**, buy new clothes that'd fit you only if you lose weight, get a bike, swimming membership, etc. . . .
Commit to something that will drive you to take action, deepen your commitment as a whole, nutrition will help massively but if you exercise it'll definitely help since you'll appreciate shedding Every ounce of fat and would do ANYTHING to never gain it again.

Learn to cook healthy stuff, even the basics!
Avoid fried foods! Roasted / boiled veggies and meat / chicken are highly recommended!

It could be the simplest thing ever to boil some eggs, boil some sweet potatoes (slow digesting carbs unlike white potatoes).

We most of the time give ourselves excuses to grab junk food, even if you never cooked anything your entire life, you can do it, there are countless of videos for free right now on Youtube that will teach you how to cook the basic stuff!

You can even go for advanced meals if you want!

Just in case you're running late sometime in the future!

Get to know the healthiest restaurants in your area, check reviews online or ask your friends / family members. I strongly recommend looking this up online!

Please, keep an open mind, keep reading and growing as a person, keep researching and coming up with better choices!

Summary of Chapter 4

- Make sure there is the least possible amount of unhealthy junk sugary foods in your house.

- That includes your fridge and all of the closets.

- No soft drinks, no frozen pizzas, no chocolate, etc.
- Get the better healthier alternative, experiment with what you like best.
- Eat a lot of green vegetables
- Get in the gym and **commit to more**
- Learn to cook healthy stuff
- Avoid fried foods

Final Word

"Success consists of going from failure to failure without loss of enthusiasm."
- Winston Churchill

First of all I want to thank you for taking your time to purchase and read this book.

If you find this book helpful and worth the value you've purchased it for, please do leave an accurate feedback of the book, this will help me improving the book and it will reaching more people as well as helping others deciding whether they find it to be the right one for them.

For more helpful content and books check out my kindle store.

I truly hope you'll take action on the instructions advised in the book as well as you sharing it with others who are struggling with this kind of addiction. It's been a pleasure serving you and providing you with what's necessary for you to grow and expand beyond your current limits and challenges.

Take action and live the life you truly deserve, it's simple, it's not easy changing your life, it takes dedication, if you're meant to succeed, you will, because the mind translates your values and standards into a reality.

Copyright

Respective authors own all copyrights not held by the publisher.

The information herein is offered for informational purposes solely, and is universal as so. The presentation of the information is without contract or any type of guarantee assurance.

The trademarks that are used are without any consent, and the publication of the trademark is without permission of backing by the trademark owner. All trademarks and brands within the book are for clarifying purposes only and are owned by the owners themselves, not affiliated with this document.

www.ingramcontent.com/pod-product-compliance
Lightning Source LLC
Chambersburg PA
CBHW070258300526
45791CB00022B/1639